BEGINNER'S BODYBUILDING

A Step-By-Step Guide to Bodybuilding Muscle and Strength

Ronald L. Abrams

BEGINNER'S BODYBUILDING

BEGINNER'S BODYBUILDING

Table Of Contents

BEGINNER'S BODYBUILDING

BEGINNER'S BODYBUILDING

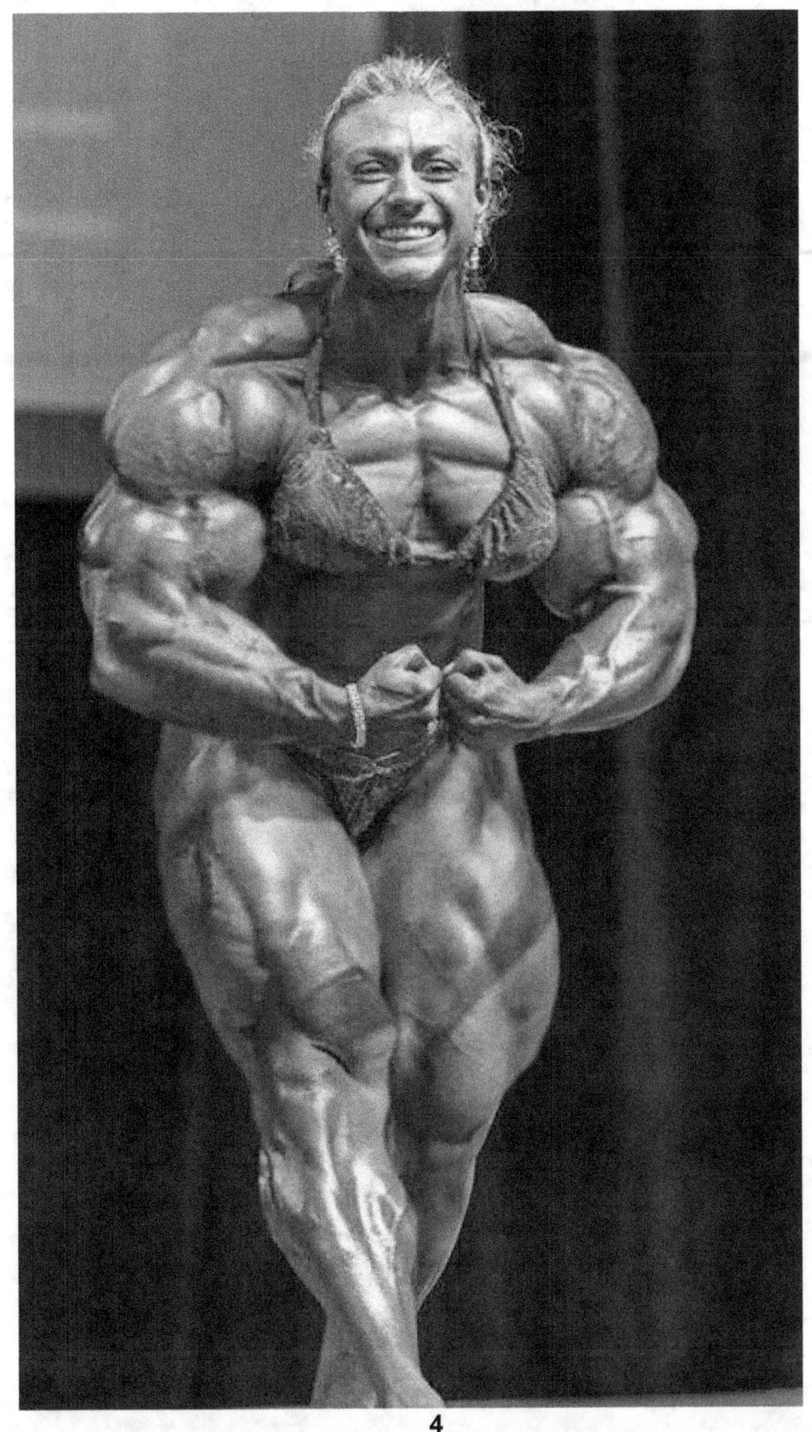

BEGINNER'S BODYBUILDING

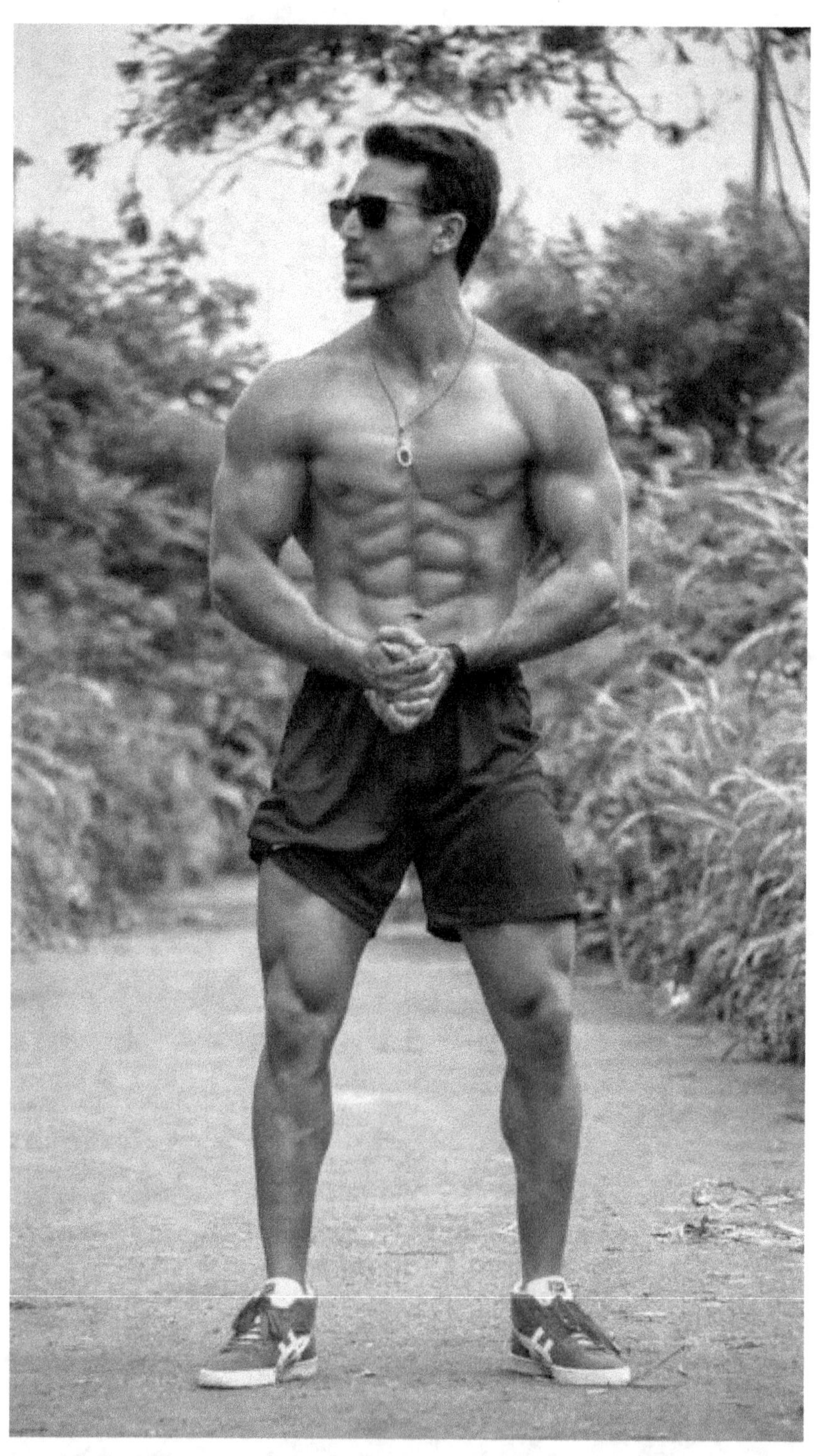

BEGINNER'S BODYBUILDING

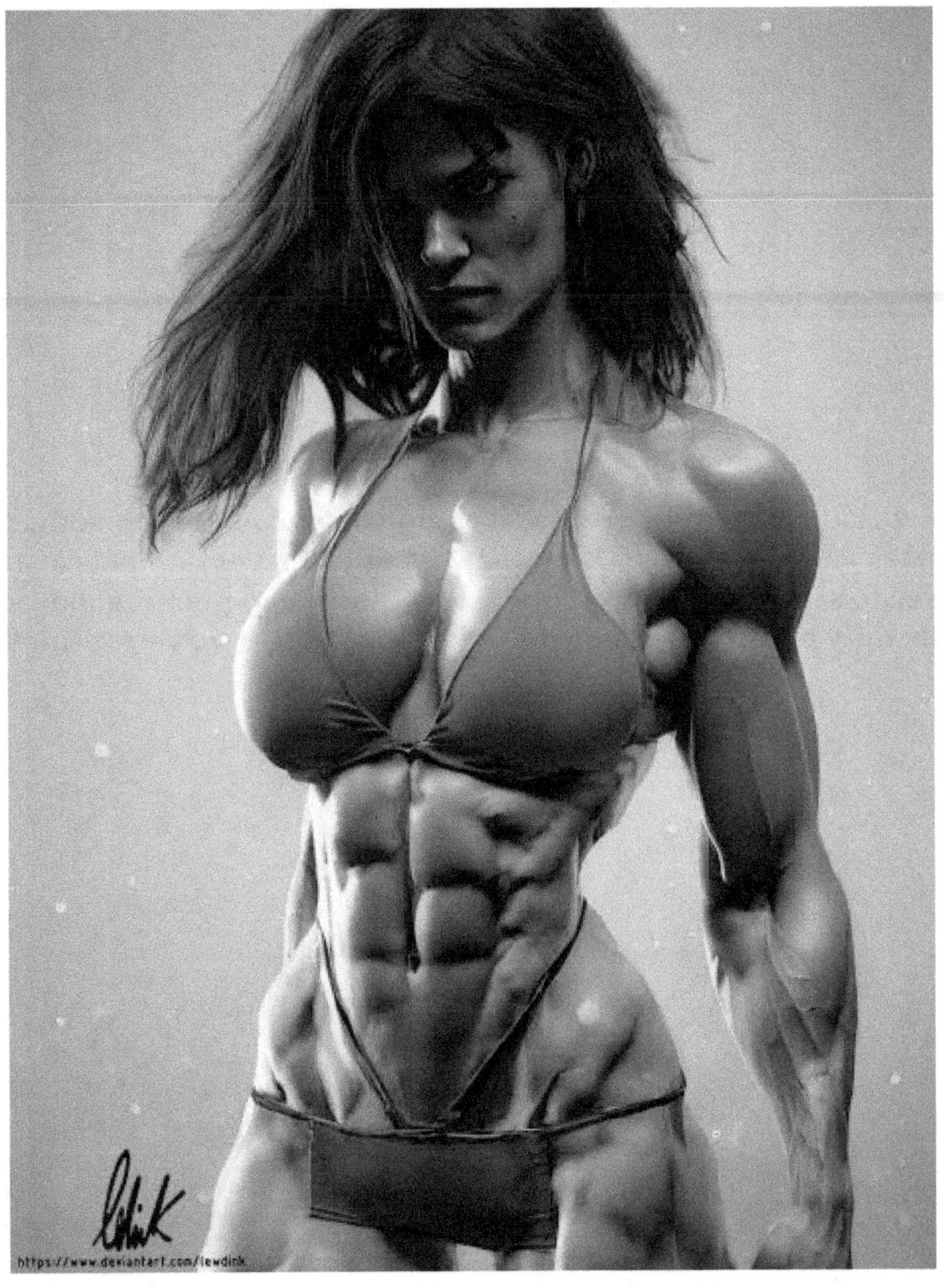

BEGINNER'S BODYBUILDING

Let that pictures of greatness you just saw be the spark that ignites your inner fire. Every lift, every rep, every meal is a step closer to sculpting your own masterpiece. Keep pushing, because the only limit is the one you set for yourself. You've got this!"

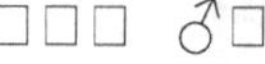

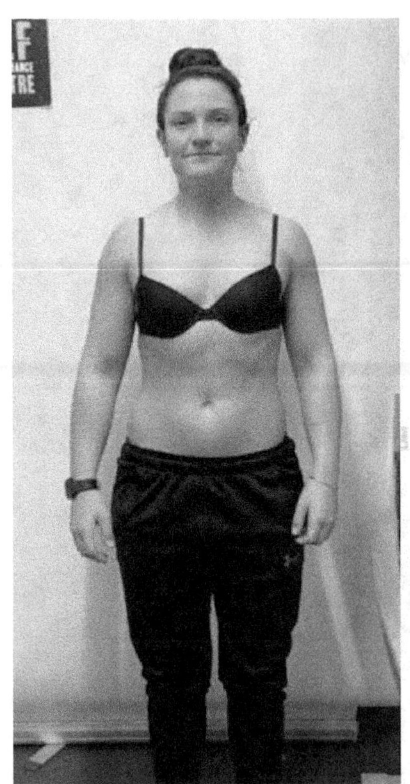

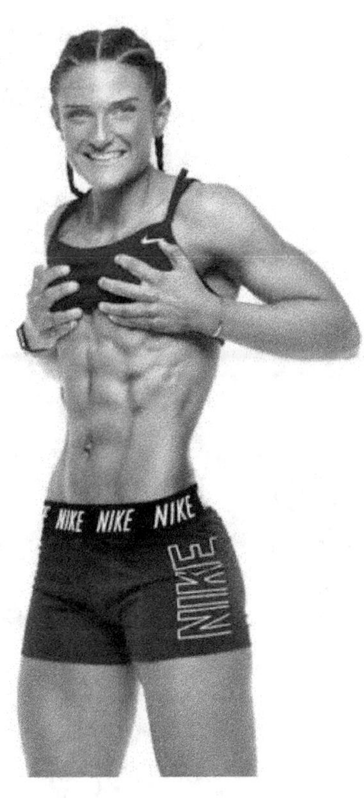

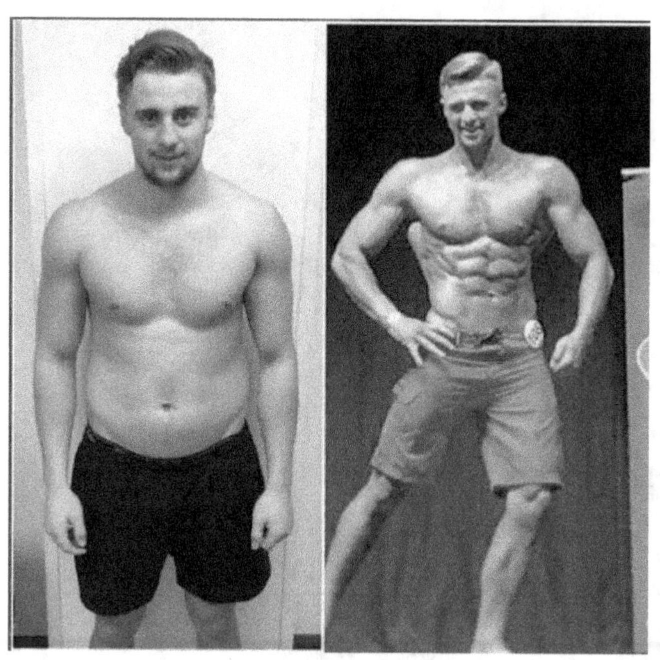

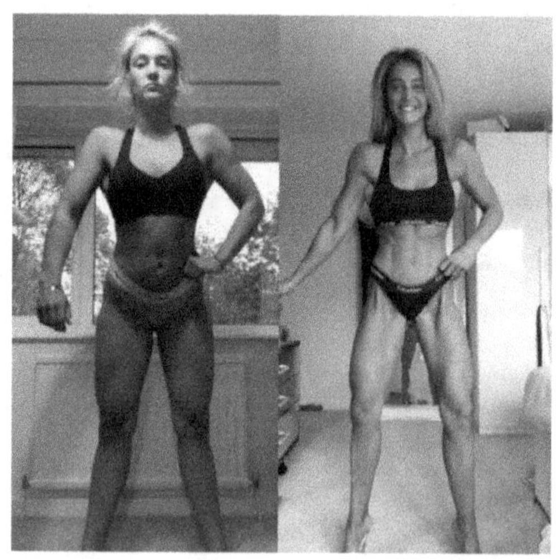

BEGINNER'S BODYBUILDING

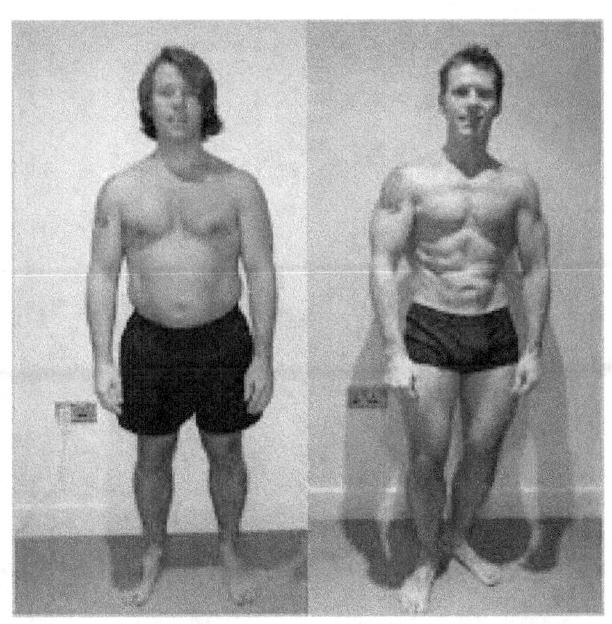

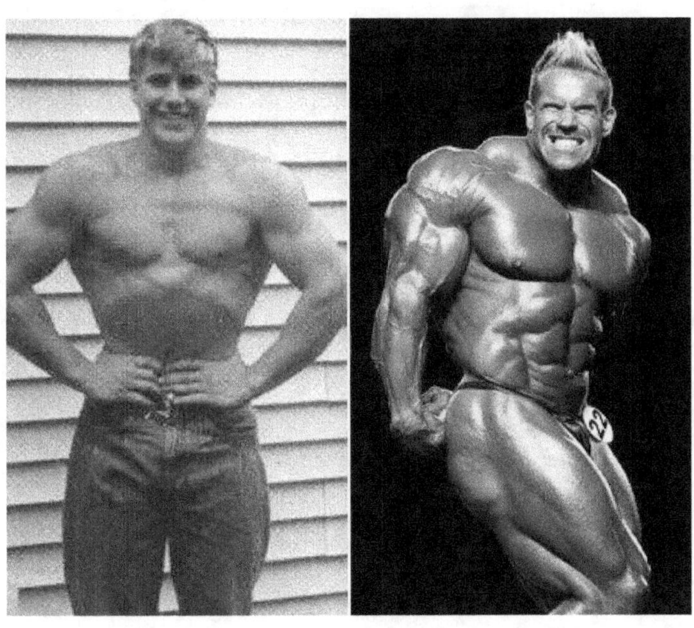

BEGINNER'S BODYBUILDING

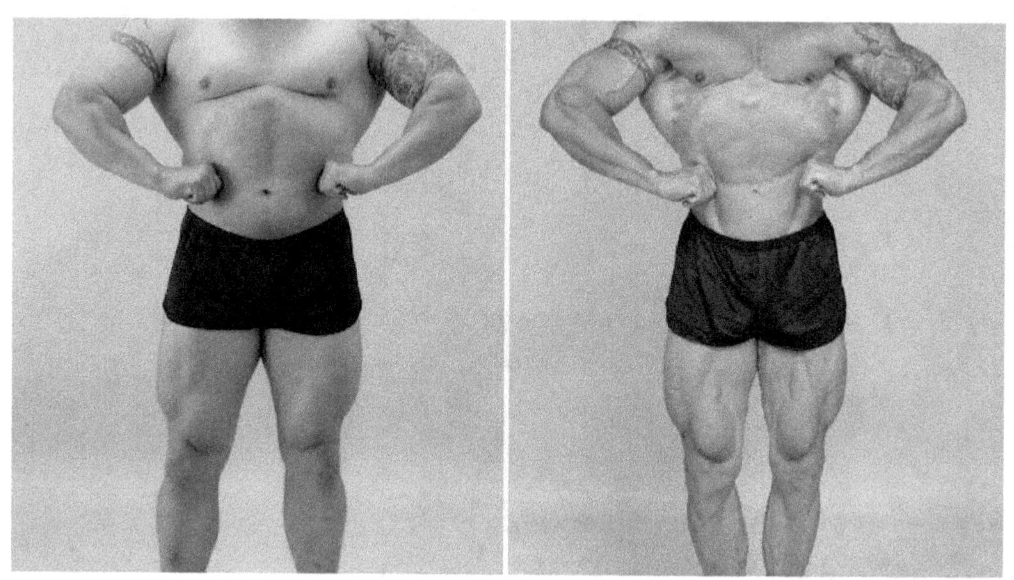

BEGINNER'S BODYBUILDING

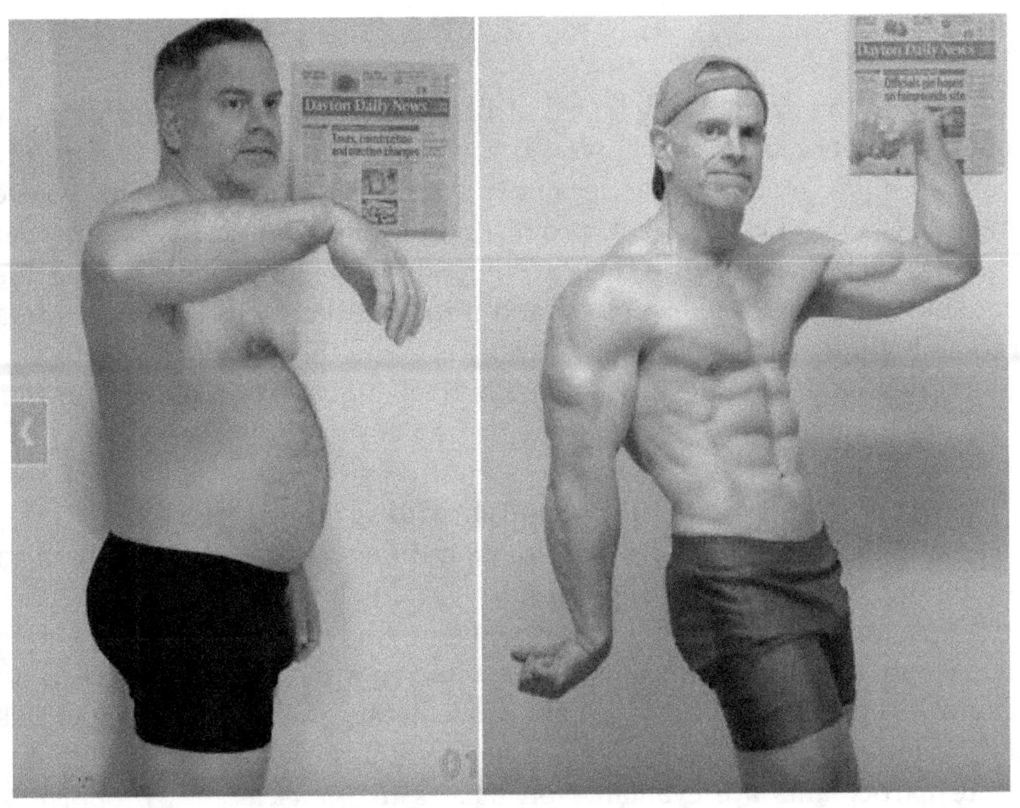

Do you want to change the way you look?
This book is exclusively for you.

BEGINNER'S BODYBUILDING

Introduction

Welcome to the exhilarating world of Beginner's Bodybuilding, where raw potential meets sculpted greatness! If you've ever dreamed of transforming your physique, building muscle, and unleashing your inner titan, you've embarked on a journey that promises not only physical strength but boundless self-discovery. In this thrilling odyssey, I guide you through the fundamental principles, exercises, and nutrition that will forge you into a true embodiment of power and grace. Get ready to unlock the secrets of your body, sculpt your destiny, and embark on a quest for the ultimate you. Welcome to the first chapter of your epic transformation!

What Is Bodybuilding?

Bodybuilding is a form of physical fitness training and sport that focuses on developing and sculpting the muscles of the body through resistance exercises, weightlifting, and a specialized diet. Bodybuilders typically aim to increase muscle size, definition, and symmetry while reducing body fat to achieve a highly muscular and aesthetic physique. Competitive bodybuilding involves showcasing these physiques in judged competitions, where participants are evaluated on factors like muscle size, proportion, and overall presentation. Bodybuilding also emphasizes discipline, nutrition, and dedication to achieve desired results.

Benefits of Bodybuilding

Benefits are advantages, rewards, or positive outcomes that individuals or entities receive as a result of a particular action, decision, program, or situation. Benefits can be financial, social, physical, emotional, or in various other forms, and they often serve as incentives or reasons for people to engage in specific activities or make certain choices.

Examples of benefits include improved health, increased income, enhanced job satisfaction, and better quality of life.

BEGINNER'S BODYBUILDING

Bodybuilding offers several benefits, including:

- Muscle development: Bodybuilding helps you build and strengthen your muscles, leading to improved physical strength and endurance.

- Improved metabolism: Building muscle can boost your metabolism, making it easier to manage your weight and body composition.

- Increased bone density: Resistance training in bodybuilding can enhance bone density, reducing the risk of osteoporosis.

- Enhanced physique: Bodybuilding can help you achieve a more sculpted and aesthetically pleasing physique.

- Better overall health: Regular exercise, including bodybuilding, can reduce the risk of chronic diseases like heart disease, diabetes, and obesity.

- Increased self-confidence: Achieving fitness goals and improving your body can boost self-esteem and self-confidence.

- Stress reduction: Exercise releases endorphins, which can help reduce stress and improve mental well-being.

- Discipline and dedication: Bodybuilding requires commitment and discipline, which can transfer to other areas of life.

- Social connections: Engaging in bodybuilding often involves joining a community of like-minded individuals who can provide support and motivation.

BEGINNER'S BODYBUILDING

- Functional strength: Building muscle can improve your ability to perform everyday tasks and reduce the risk of injury.

It's important to approach bodybuilding with proper technique, nutrition, and rest to maximize these benefits and minimize the risk of injury. Consulting with a fitness professional or trainer can be helpful for beginners.

BEGINNER'S BODYBUILDING

Chapter 1

SETTING YOUR GOALS

Setting goals is like embarking on a journey; the destination represents your desired outcome, and the path you take defines your strategy.

Setting effective bodybuilding goals is crucial for achieving success in your fitness journey. These goals provide direction, motivation, and a sense of purpose to your workouts. To begin, it's essential to establish clear and specific objectives. These could include gaining muscle mass, reducing body fat, improving strength, or enhancing overall fitness.

Here's a vivid explanation of setting goals:

1. Choose Your Destination: Imagine standing at a crossroads in a vast forest. Your first step is to decide where you want to go. Your destination should be clear, specific, and inspiring. It's like selecting a hidden treasure deep within the forest, motivating you to navigate through the challenges.

2. Define the Path: Once you know your destination, you must chart your course. Think of this as creating a detailed map with markers along the way. These markers represent milestones or smaller goals that will guide you and help you stay on track.

3. Set SMART Goals: Your goals should be SMART: Specific, Measurable, Achievable, Relevant, and Time-bound. This ensures they are well-defined and realistic. It's like plotting the exact coordinates of your treasure on the map, making it easier to follow.

4. Visualize Success: Close your eyes and picture yourself reaching your goal. Imagine the emotions, the sense of accomplishment, and the

rewards that come with it. This mental image is like the beacon of light guiding you through the forest.

5. Break it Down: Goals can be overwhelming, so break them down into smaller, manageable tasks. These tasks are like stepping stones in your journey, each taking you closer to your destination.

6. Stay Committed: Just as a hiker perseveres through rain and rough terrain, commitment is essential. Maintain focus, remind yourself of your vision, and don't be discouraged by setbacks.

7. Track Progress: Regularly check your map and assess how far you've come. Celebrate your achievements, and if you've deviated from your path, recalibrate and adjust your goals as needed.

8. Seek Support: Share your goals with trusted friends or mentors who can provide guidance and motivation. They can be like fellow travelers who share wisdom from their own journeys.

9. Adaptability: Be prepared to adapt to unforeseen circumstances or changes in your priorities. Think of this as taking detours or switching trails when necessary, while still keeping your final destination in mind.

10. Enjoy the Journey: Lastly, remember that the journey itself is as important as the destination. Embrace the experiences, learn from them, and savor the growth you achieve along the way.

In essence, setting goals is about creating a roadmap for your aspirations, ensuring you have a clear vision of where you're headed and the determination to reach that elusive treasure at the end of your journey.

BEGINNER'S BODYBUILDING

Defining Your Fitness Goals

Defining your fitness goals is a crucial first step in creating a personalized fitness plan. To do this, consider the following:

1. Specificity: Clearly define what you want to achieve. Do you want to lose weight, build muscle, increase endurance, or improve flexibility?

2. Measurable: Set quantifiable goals. For example, aim to lose a certain number of pounds, lift a specific weight, or run a particular distance.

3. Achievable: Ensure your goals are realistic and attainable within your current circumstances, such as your time, resources, and fitness level.

4. Relevant: Make sure your goals align with your overall health and well-being. They should be meaningful to you.

5. Time-bound: Set a deadline or timeframe for achieving your goals. This adds urgency and helps you stay motivated.

6. Adaptability: Be willing to adjust your goals as needed based on your progress and changing circumstances.

7. Consult a professional: Consider seeking guidance from a fitness trainer or healthcare provider to help you set appropriate and safe goals.

Remember that fitness goals should be tailored to your individual needs and preferences. They can evolve over time as you make progress and discover what works best for you.

BEGINNER'S BODYBUILDING

Realistic Expectations

Realistic Expectations in bodybuilding depend on various factors including genetics, training consistency, nutrition, and goals. It's important to:

- Set achievable short-term and long-term goals.

- Understand that progress takes time, often years.

- Recognize genetic limitations and focus on personal improvement.

- Prioritize safety over rapid gains to avoid injuries.

- Embrace the journey and enjoy the process of self-improvement.

Note; Consulting with a fitness professional can help tailor expectations to your specific circumstances and goals.

BEGINNER'S BODYBUILDING

Chapter 2

NUTRITION FOR BODYBUILDING

Nutrition is a critical component of bodybuilding, as it plays a pivotal role in helping individuals achieve their fitness goals. Proper nutrition provides the body with the essential nutrients, energy, and support needed for muscle growth, repair, and overall performance. In this context, I'll delve into the key aspects of nutrition for bodybuilding, including macronutrients, micronutrients, meal timing, and dietary strategies that optimize muscle development and recovery.

Proper nutrition is crucial for bodybuilders for several reasons:

- Muscle Growth: Adequate protein intake is essential to repair and build muscle tissue after workouts.

- Energy: Carbohydrates provide the energy needed for intense training sessions.

- Recovery: Nutrients like vitamins, minerals, and antioxidants aid in recovery and reduce muscle soreness.

- Body Composition: Proper nutrition helps control body fat levels and maintain a lean physique.

- Hormone Regulation: Nutrient balance influences hormone levels, affecting muscle growth and fat loss.

- Immune Function: Good nutrition supports a strong immune system, reducing the risk of illness that could hinder training.

BEGINNER'S BODYBUILDING

- Performance: Optimal nutrition enhances strength, endurance, and overall athletic performance.

- Injury Prevention: Nutrients like calcium and vitamin D support bone health, reducing the risk of fractures.

- Mental Focus: Balanced nutrition can improve mental clarity and concentration during workouts.

- Longevity: A healthy diet can help bodybuilders maintain their physique and overall health as they age.

In summary, proper nutrition is the foundation of success for bodybuilders, supporting muscle growth, performance, recovery, and overall health.

Micronutrients

Macronutrients are essential nutrients that provide energy and are required in relatively large amounts by the human body. There are three primary macronutrients:

Carbohydrates: These are the body's primary source of energy and include sugars, starches, and fiber. Good sources of carbohydrates include grains, fruits, vegetables, and legumes.

Carbohydrates are an important source of energy for bodybuilders. Here's a list of carbohydrate-rich foods suitable for bodybuilders:

1. Complex Carbohydrates:
- Brown rice
- Quinoa
- Oats

BEGINNER'S BODYBUILDING

- Sweet potatoes
- Whole wheat pasta
- Whole grain bread

2. Fruits:
- Bananas
- Apples
- Berries (strawberries, blueberries, raspberries)
- Oranges
- Pineapple

3. Vegetables:
- Broccoli
- Spinach
- Kale
- Carrots
- Bell peppers

4. Legumes:
- Chickpeas
- Lentils
- Black beans
- Kidney beans

5. Dairy and Dairy Alternatives:
- Greek yogurt
- Milk (or almond, soy, or coconut milk)
- Cottage cheese

6. Grains and Cereals:
- Whole grain cereal

BEGINNER'S BODYBUILDING

- Granola
- Barley

7. Snacks:
- Popcorn (air-popped)
- Rice cakes
- Whole grain crackers

8. Energy Bars:
- Look for bars with oats, nuts, and dried fruits

Remember that a balanced diet is key for bodybuilders, so these carbohydrates should be part of a well-rounded nutrition plan that includes protein and healthy fats to support muscle growth and recovery. Consult with a nutritionist or dietitian for personalized guidance.

Proteins: Proteins are essential for building and repairing tissues, and they also play a role in various bodily functions. Sources of protein include meat, fish, poultry, dairy products, beans, and tofu.

Protein is essential for bodybuilders to support muscle growth and repair. Here's a list of protein-rich foods for bodybuilders:

1. Chicken breast
2. Turkey
3. Lean beef
4. Salmon
5. Tuna
6. Eggs
7. Greek yogurt
8. Cottage cheese

BEGINNER'S BODYBUILDING

9. Tofu
10.   Lentils
11. Chickpeas
12. Quinoa
13. Edamame
14. Peanut butter
15. Whey protein powder

These foods provide a variety of protein sources, including animal and plant-based options, to help meet the protein needs of bodybuilders. Remember to balance your protein intake with carbohydrates and healthy fats for a well-rounded diet.

Remember to balance protein intake with carbohydrates and healthy fats for a well-rounded diet to support your fitness goals.

Fats: Fats are another source of energy and are important for overall health. They are categorized into saturated fats, unsaturated fats, and trans fats. Sources of healthy fats include avocados, nuts, seeds, and olive oil.

Bodybuilders often include healthy fats in their diets to support muscle growth and overall health. Here's a list of fats that can be beneficial for bodybuilders:

1. Avocado: Rich in monounsaturated fats, avocados provide healthy calories and various vitamins and minerals.

2. Nuts and seeds: Almonds, walnuts, chia seeds, and flaxseeds are good sources of healthy fats, protein, and fiber.

BEGINNER'S BODYBUILDING

3. Fatty fish: Salmon, mackerel, and trout contain omega-3 fatty acids, which have anti-inflammatory properties and support muscle recovery.

4. Olive oil: Extra virgin olive oil is high in monounsaturated fats and can be used for cooking or as a salad dressing.

5. Nut butters: Peanut butter, almond butter, and cashew butter offer healthy fats and protein.

6. Coconut oil: This oil contains medium-chain triglycerides (MCTs) that can provide a quick source of energy.

7. Eggs: The yolks are rich in healthy fats, vitamins, and minerals, making them a great addition to a bodybuilder's diet.

8. Dark chocolate: In moderation, dark chocolate with a high cocoa content can provide antioxidants and healthy fats.

9. Cheese: Options like feta, cottage cheese, and some hard cheeses are high in protein and healthy fats.

10. Grass-fed butter: It contains omega-3 fatty acids and conjugated linoleic acid (CLA), which can be beneficial.

Remember that portion control and overall calorie intake are important factors for bodybuilders, so while these fats are beneficial, they should be consumed in moderation as part of a well-balanced diet.

Balancing these macronutrients in your diet is crucial for maintaining good health and energy levels. The specific proportions of macronutrients you

BEGINNER'S BODYBUILDING

need may vary based on factors like age, gender, activity level, and individual health goals.

Micronutrients

Micronutrients are essential nutrients that our body requires in smaller quantities compared to macronutrients like carbohydrates, proteins, and fats. They include vitamins and minerals, which play crucial roles in various bodily functions. Micronutrients are essential for maintaining good health, supporting metabolism, and preventing deficiencies or diseases. Examples of micronutrients include vitamins such as vitamin A, vitamin C, and minerals like iron, calcium, and zinc. A balanced diet that includes a variety of foods can help ensure you get an adequate intake of these micronutrients.

Vitamins

Bodybuilders often focus on specific vitamins and minerals to support their training and overall health. Some key vitamins and minerals for bodybuilders include:

1. Vitamin D: Supports bone health and muscle function. Bodybuilders often need sufficient Vitamin D for muscle health and overall well-being. Foods rich in Vitamin D include:

- Fatty fish like salmon, mackerel, and tuna.
- Fortified dairy products like milk and yogurt.
- Egg yolks.
- Beef liver.
- Cheese (especially Swiss and cheddar).
- Fortified cereals and orange juice.
- Mushrooms (if exposed to sunlight).

BEGINNER'S BODYBUILDING

However, it can be challenging to meet Vitamin D needs through diet alone, so consider getting sunlight exposure and consulting a healthcare professional or dietitian for personalized advice or supplements if necessary.

2. Vitamin C: Helps with collagen production and immune support.
Vitamin C is important for everyone, including bodybuilders, as it plays a role in overall health and can support exercise recovery. While it doesn't directly build muscle, it does have several benefits for bodybuilders:

- Immune Support: Intense training can stress the immune system. Vitamin C is known for its immune-boosting properties, helping to keep you healthy and training consistently.

- Collagen Production: Vitamin C is essential for collagen synthesis, which is crucial for maintaining healthy tendons, ligaments, and skin. This can be particularly important for bodybuilders who put extra strain on these tissues.

- Antioxidant Protection: Vitamin C is a potent antioxidant that helps combat oxidative stress caused by intense workouts. This can aid in reducing muscle soreness and inflammation.

- Iron Absorption: It aids in the absorption of non-heme iron (found in plant-based foods), which is important for preventing iron deficiency anemia in individuals with vegetarian or vegan diets.

To incorporate vitamin C into your diet, include foods like citrus fruits (oranges, lemons), berries (strawberries, blueberries), kiwi, peppers (red and green), and broccoli. A balanced diet with a variety of nutrients is essential for bodybuilders to support their training and recovery.

3. Vitamin B complex: Includes B1 (thiamine), B2 (riboflavin), B3 (niacin), B6 (pyridoxine), and B12 (cobalamin), which play a role in energy metabolism.

Vitamin B is important for energy metabolism, which is crucial for bodybuilders. Foods rich in various B vitamins include:

- B1 (Thiamine): Whole grains, lean pork, and nuts.
- B2 (Riboflavin): Dairy products, lean meats, and green leafy vegetables.
- B3 (Niacin): Chicken, turkey, salmon, and peanuts.
- B5 (Pantothenic Acid): Eggs, avocados, and whole grains.
- B6 (Pyridoxine): Bananas, chickpeas, and lean beef.
- B7 (Biotin): Eggs, nuts, and sweet potatoes.
- B9 (Folate): Leafy greens, beans, and fortified cereals.
- B12 (Cobalamin): Meat, fish, and dairy products.

Incorporating these foods into your diet can help support your energy levels and overall health as a bodybuilder. However, remember that supplements should be considered only if you have a deficiency, and it's best to consult a healthcare professional for personalized advice.

4. Vitamin A: Important for vision and immune function.

Vitamin A is important for bodybuilders as it supports various functions, including immune system health and vision. Good sources of vitamin A for bodybuilders include:

BEGINNER'S BODYBUILDING

- Sweet potatoes
- Carrots
- Spinach
- Kale
- Broccoli
- Bell peppers
- Mangoes
- Apricots
- Eggs (specifically the yolk)
- Liver (in moderation)

Incorporating these foods into your diet can help you maintain optimal health while pursuing your bodybuilding goals.

5. Vitamin E: Acts as an antioxidant to protect cells from damage.

Vitamin E is important for bodybuilders as it helps protect cells from oxidative damage, which can occur during intense workouts. Some vitamin E-rich foods for bodybuilders include:

- Nuts and Seeds (e.g., almonds, sunflower seeds)
- Spinach and Other Leafy Greens
- Avocado
- Whole Grains (e.g., wheat germ)
- Fish (e.g., salmon)
- Vegetable Oils (e.g., sunflower oil)
- Kiwi
- Mangoes

Incorporating these foods into your diet can help you meet your vitamin E needs as a bodybuilder. Remember to maintain a balanced diet to support overall muscle growth and recovery.

6. Calcium: Essential for muscle contractions and bone health.

Calcium is important for maintaining strong bones and muscles, which is essential for bodybuilders. Here is a list of calcium-rich foods suitable for bodybuilders:

1. Dairy Products:
- Milk
- Yogurt
- Cheese

2. Leafy Greens:
- Spinach
- Kale
- Collard greens

3. Fortified Foods:
- Fortified plant-based milk (e.g., almond milk, soy milk)
- Fortified orange juice

4. Canned Fish with Bones:
- Sardines
- Salmon (with bones)

5. Tofu:
- Firm tofu is often fortified with calcium.

6. Nuts and Seeds:
- Almonds

BEGINNER'S BODYBUILDING

- Chia seeds

7. Legumes:
- White beans
- Chickpeas
- Broccoli
8. Figs (dried)
9. Oranges

Including a variety of these foods in your diet can help ensure you get an adequate amount of calcium as a bodybuilder. Remember to balance calcium intake with other essential nutrients for overall health and muscle function.

7. Magnesium: Supports muscle and nerve function, as well as energy production.

Here is a list of magnesium-rich foods that can be beneficial for bodybuilders:

- Spinach
- Almonds
- Pumpkin seeds
- Avocado
- Black beans
- Brown rice
- Tofu
- Salmon
- Bananas
- Whole wheat bread
- Cashews
- Quinoa

BEGINNER'S BODYBUILDING

- Yogurt
- Dark chocolate (in moderation)
- Edamame
- Sunflower seeds
- Oatmeal
- Chickpeas
- Brazil nuts
- Mackerel

Including these foods in your diet can help ensure you get an adequate intake of magnesium, which is important for muscle function and overall health for bodybuilders.

8. Zinc: Aids in muscle recovery and immune function.

Zinc is an essential mineral for bodybuilders as it plays a role in muscle growth and overall health. Here are some zinc-rich foods suitable for bodybuilders:

- Lean meats (beef, chicken, turkey)
- Seafood (oysters, crab, lobster, shrimp)
- Dairy products (cheese, yogurt)
- Eggs
- Nuts and seeds (pumpkin seeds, cashews)
- Legumes (chickpeas, lentils)
- Whole grains (oats, quinoa)
- Dark chocolate (in moderation)
- Tofu and tempeh (for vegetarians and vegans)

Incorporating these zinc-rich foods into your diet can help support muscle growth and overall performance as a bodybuilder. Remember to maintain a balanced diet for optimal results.

BEGINNER'S BODYBUILDING

9. Iron: Necessary for oxygen transport in the blood.
Iron is an important mineral for bodybuilders as it helps transport oxygen to muscles. Here are some iron-rich foods suitable for bodybuilders:

- Lean red meat (beef, pork, lamb)
- Poultry (chicken, turkey)
- Fish (salmon, tuna, sardines)
- Lean cuts of beef (such as sirloin or tenderloin)
- Eggs (especially egg yolks)
- Legumes (beans, lentils, chickpeas)
- Tofu and tempeh
- Spinach and other dark leafy greens
- Fortified cereals
- Nuts and seeds (especially pumpkin seeds)
- Quinoa
- Dried fruits (like apricots and raisins)

Incorporating a variety of these iron-rich foods into your diet can help ensure you meet your iron needs as a bodybuilder.

Remember to balance iron intake with other essential nutrients for a well-rounded diet. Consult a healthcare professional or nutritionist for personalized guidance.

It's essential for bodybuilders to maintain a well-balanced diet to ensure they get these nutrients. However, individual needs may vary, so consulting with a healthcare professional or nutritionist can help tailor a vitamin and mineral regimen to specific goals and requirements. Additionally, supplements should be used cautiously and as directed to avoid excessive intake.

Meal Planning and Timing

BEGINNER'S BODYBUILDING

Meal planning and timing are essential aspects of maintaining a healthy and balanced lifestyle. In today's fast-paced world, where convenience often takes precedence, thoughtful meal planning and timing can make a significant difference in our overall well-being. These practices involve not only deciding what to eat but also when to eat it, ensuring that our bodies receive the necessary nutrients at the right times. In this discussion, we will delve into the importance of meal planning and timing, exploring how they can positively impact our health, energy levels, and overall quality of life. Whether you're looking to manage your weight, boost your metabolism, or simply make better food choices, understanding the principles of meal planning and timing is a valuable step towards achieving your health and nutrition goals.

Bodybuilders often follow a structured meal plan and timing strategy to support their muscle growth and overall fitness goals. Here are some key considerations:

1. Protein Intake: Protein is essential for muscle repair and growth. Bodybuilders typically consume protein-rich foods like lean meats, poultry, fish, eggs, dairy, and plant-based sources like tofu and legumes. Aim for a consistent intake of protein throughout the day.

2. Meal Frequency: Many bodybuilders prefer to eat 5-6 smaller meals a day to maintain a steady supply of nutrients for muscle recovery and energy.

3. Carbohydrates: Carbohydrates provide energy for workouts and replenish glycogen stores. Complex carbohydrates like whole grains, oats, and sweet potatoes are favored over simple sugars.

BEGINNER'S BODYBUILDING

4. Healthy Fats: Include sources of healthy fats like avocados, nuts, seeds, and olive oil to support overall health and hormone balance.

5. Pre-Workout Nutrition: Consume a balanced meal with carbohydrates and protein about 1-2 hours before a workout to provide energy and support muscle function.

6. Post-Workout Nutrition: After a workout, have a meal or shake with both protein and carbohydrates to aid in muscle recovery and glycogen replenishment.

7. Meal Timing: Timing can be crucial. Some bodybuilders emphasize nutrient timing, such as consuming fast-digesting protein and carbs immediately after a workout.

8. Hydration: Staying hydrated is essential for performance and recovery. Drink water throughout the day, and consider electrolyte-rich beverages during intense workouts.

9. Supplements: Some bodybuilders use supplements like protein powder, creatine, and branched-chain amino acids (BCAAs) to support their nutrition.

10. Caloric Surplus or Deficit: Adjust your calorie intake based on your goals. To build muscle, a slight caloric surplus may be needed, while fat loss requires a caloric deficit.

11. Rest and Sleep: Ensure you get enough rest and quality sleep, as this is when muscle recovery and growth occur.

BEGINNER'S BODYBUILDING

12. Individualized Plan: Meal plans should be tailored to individual preferences, dietary restrictions, and goals. Consulting with a registered dietitian or nutritionist can be beneficial.

Remember that consistency is key in bodybuilding nutrition. It's important to monitor progress and adjust your plan as needed to meet your specific goals. Always consult with a healthcare professional or nutrition expert before making significant dietary changes or taking supplements.

A 7 Day Meal Plann and Timing

A 7-day meal plan for a beginner's bodybuilding workout routine should focus on providing enough protein, carbohydrates, and healthy fats to support muscle growth and recovery. Here's a sample meal plan with approximate timings:

Day 1 - Monday:

1. **Breakfast (7:00 AM):** Scrambled eggs with spinach and whole-grain toast.
2. **Snack (10:00 AM):** Greek yogurt with berries and honey.
3. **Lunch (1:00 PM):** Grilled chicken breast, quinoa, and steamed broccoli.
4. **Pre-workout (4:00 PM):** A banana and a handful of almonds.
5. **Dinner (7:00 PM):** Baked salmon, sweet potato, and mixed vegetables.

Day 2 - Tuesday:

1. **Breakfast (7:00 AM):** Oatmeal with protein powder, almond butter, and banana slices.
2. **Snack (10:00 AM):** Cottage cheese with pineapple.

BEGINNER'S BODYBUILDING

3. **Lunch (1:00 PM):** Lean ground turkey with brown rice and asparagus.
4. **Pre-workout (4:00 PM):** Whole-grain crackers with hummus.
5. **Dinner (7:00 PM):** Grilled shrimp, quinoa, and roasted Brussels sprouts.

Day 3 - Wednesday:

1. **Breakfast (7:00 AM):** Whole-grain pancakes with blueberries and a side of scrambled eggs.
2. **Snack (10:00 AM):** Mixed nuts and dried fruits.
3. **Lunch (1:00 PM):** Grilled chicken breast with mixed greens and olive oil dressing.
4. **Pre-workout (4:00 PM):** Greek yogurt with sliced almonds.
5. **Dinner (7:00 PM):** Lean beef stir-fry with brown rice and broccoli.

Day 4 - Thursday:

1. **Breakfast (7:00 AM):** Protein smoothie with spinach, banana, and whey protein.
2. **Snack (10:00 AM):** Sliced apples with peanut butter.
3. **Lunch (1:00 PM):** Baked tilapia, quinoa, and steamed green beans.
4. **Pre-workout (4:00 PM):** Carrots and hummus.
5. **Dinner (7:00 PM):** Turkey meatballs with whole-grain pasta and tomato sauce.

Day 5 - Friday:

1. **Breakfast (7:00 AM):** Scrambled eggs with diced tomatoes and avocado.
2. **Snack (10:00 AM):** Low-fat cottage cheese with sliced peaches.

BEGINNER'S BODYBUILDING

3. **Lunch (1:00 PM)**: Grilled chicken breast, brown rice, and mixed vegetables.
4. **Pre-workout (4:00 PM)**: A protein bar.
5. **Dinner (7:00 PM)**: Baked cod with quinoa and sautéed spinach.

Day 6 - Saturday:

1. **Breakfast (7:00 AM)**: Protein-rich smoothie with berries, spinach, and almond milk.
2. **Snack (10:00 AM):** Sliced cucumber with hummus.
3. **Lunch (1:00 PM)**: Lean beef steak, sweet potato, and asparagus.
4. **Pre-workout (4:00 PM)**: Greek yogurt with honey.
5. **Dinner (7:00 PM):** Grilled chicken breast, brown rice, and roasted carrots.

Day 7 - Sunday (Rest Day):

1. **Breakfast (8:00 AM)**: Whole-grain waffles with maple syrup and a side of Greek yogurt.
2. **Snack (11:00 AM)**: Mixed nuts and a protein shake.
3. **Lunch (2:00 PM)**: Turkey and avocado sandwich on whole-grain bread with a side salad.
4. **Snack (5:00 PM)**: A piece of fruit.
5. **Dinner (8:00 PM)**: Baked salmon, quinoa, and steamed broccoli.

Don't forget to adjust portion sizes and calorie intake based on your specific goals and dietary needs. It's also important to stay hydrated throughout the day and consult with a nutritionist or dietitian for a personalized meal plan tailored to your needs and goals.

BEGINNER'S BODYBUILDING

Chapter 3

RESISTANT TRAINING

Resistance training, also known as strength or weight training, is a form of exercise designed to improve muscular strength, endurance, and overall fitness. It involves the use of external resistance, such as dumbbells, barbells, resistance bands, or even one's body weight, to create resistance against muscle contraction. This type of training is not only popular among athletes and bodybuilders but also provides numerous health benefits for people of all fitness levels. In this conversation, we can explore the principles, techniques, and advantages of resistance training in more detail.

Understanding Resistant Training.

Resistance training, also known as strength or weight training, is a type of exercise that involves using resistance to build and strengthen muscles. Here are some key points to help you understand resistance training:

1. Purpose: The primary goal of resistance training is to increase muscular strength, endurance, and size. It can also improve overall fitness and help with weight management.

2. Resistance: Resistance can come from various sources, including free weights (dumbbells and barbells), machines, resistance bands, or even your body weight. The resistance creates tension in the muscles, leading to adaptation and growth.

3. Types of Exercises: Common resistance training exercises include squats, bench presses, deadlifts, bicep curls, and push-ups, among others. These exercises target specific muscle groups.

BEGINNER'S BODYBUILDING

4. Progressive Overload: To see improvements, you must gradually increase the resistance or intensity of your workouts. This concept is known as progressive overload and is essential for muscle growth.

5. Sets and Repetitions: Workouts are typically organized into sets (a group of repetitions) and repetitions (the number of times you perform a specific movement within a set). The number of sets and reps can vary depending on your goals.

6. Rest and Recovery: Muscles need time to recover and grow after resistance training. Adequate rest and recovery days are crucial to avoid overtraining and injuries.

7. Form and Technique: Proper form is essential to prevent injuries and maximize the effectiveness of each exercise. If you're new to resistance training, consider working with a trainer to learn the correct techniques.

8. Nutrition: A balanced diet with adequate protein is important to support muscle growth and recovery. Many people also use supplements like protein powder to help meet their nutritional needs.

9. Safety Precautions: Always warm up before starting a resistance training session, and cool down afterward. It's also important to use proper safety equipment and spotter assistance when needed, especially for heavy lifts.

10. Variety: Incorporating a variety of exercises into your routine can prevent plateaus and keep your workouts interesting. Target different muscle groups on different days.

BEGINNER'S BODYBUILDING

11. Consistency: Consistency is key to seeing results in resistance training. Aim for regular workouts and gradually increase the intensity over time.

12. Consult a Professional: If you're new to resistance training or have specific fitness goals, consider consulting a fitness professional or personal trainer to create a customized workout plan.

Be aware that resistance training can benefit people of all ages and fitness levels, but it's important to start at an appropriate level and progress safely to avoid injuries. It's also advisable to consult with a healthcare provider before beginning any new exercise program, especially if you have preexisting medical conditions.

Basic Weightlifting Techniques

Basic weightlifting techniques are fundamental for anyone looking to build strength, improve fitness, or engage in competitive weightlifting. These techniques involve lifting weights with proper form and control to maximize results while minimizing the risk of injury. Key aspects of basic weightlifting techniques include proper body positioning, breathing, and movement patterns. Whether you're a beginner or an experienced lifter, mastering these fundamentals is essential for a safe and effective weightlifting journey. In this discussion, we'll explore some of these foundational techniques to help you get started or refine your skills in the world of weightlifting.

Basic weightlifting techniques are essential for anyone starting with weight training. Here are some fundamental techniques for common weightlifting exercises:

1. Squat:

BEGINNER'S BODYBUILDING

- Stand with your feet shoulder-width apart.
- Keep your chest up, shoulders back, and core engaged.
- Lower your body by bending at your hips and knees.
- Aim to keep your knees in line with your toes and go as low as your flexibility allows.
- Push through your heels to stand back up.

2. Deadlift:

- Stand with your feet hip-width apart and a barbell over the mid-foot.
- Bend at your hips and knees to lower your body down to the barbell.
- Grab the barbell with an overhand or mixed grip (one palm facing you, one palm facing away).
- Keep your back straight, chest up, and arms extended.
- Lift the barbell by straightening your hips and knees, pushing your hips forward.
- Lower the barbell by bending at your hips and knees with control.

3. Bench Press:

- Lie on a flat bench with your feet flat on the floor.
- Grip the barbell slightly wider than shoulder-width apart.
- Lower the barbell to your chest in a controlled manner, keeping your elbows at around a 45-degree angle.
- Push the barbell back up to the starting position, locking out your elbows.

4. Bent-Over Row:

- Stand with your feet hip-width apart and hold a barbell or dumbbells with an overhand grip.

- Bend at your hips to lean forward while keeping your back straight.
- Pull the weight toward your lower ribcage by bending your elbows and squeezing your shoulder blades together.
- Lower the weight back down with control.

5. Overhead Press (Shoulder Press):

- Stand with your feet hip-width apart.
- Hold a barbell or dumbbells at shoulder height with your palms facing forward.
- Press the weight overhead by extending your arms, without arching your lower back.
- Lower the weight back to shoulder height with control.

6. Pull-Ups:

- Hang from a pull-up bar with your palms facing away from your body.
- Engage your core and pull your body upward until your chin clears the bar.
- Lower your body back down to the starting position with control.

7. Push-Ups:

- Start in a plank position with your hands slightly wider than shoulder-width apart.
- Lower your body by bending your elbows while keeping your body in a straight line.
- Push your body back up to the starting position.

8. Lunges:

BEGINNER'S BODYBUILDING

- Stand with your feet together.
- Take a step forward with one leg and lower your body until both knees are bent at a 90-degree angle.
- Push off the front foot to return to the starting position.
- Repeat on the other leg.

Always try to use proper form, start with lighter weights, and gradually increase the weight as you become more comfortable and experienced. If you're new to weightlifting, consider working with a trainer to ensure you're using correct techniques and to prevent injuries.

Choosing The Right Exercises

Choosing the right exercises for bodybuilding is essential to maximize muscle growth and overall progress. It's a crucial aspect of any effective workout routine. In this guide, we'll explore key principles for selecting exercises that target specific muscle groups, promote balanced development, and align with your fitness goals. Whether you're a beginner or an experienced lifter, understanding how to choose the right exercises is fundamental to achieving your bodybuilding objectives.

For a beginner's bodybuilding workout, it's important to focus on building a strong foundation. Here are some exercises to consider:

1. Compound Movements:

- Squats: Great for leg and core development.
- Deadlifts: Work on your entire posterior chain.
- Bench Press: Targets chest and triceps.
- Pull-Ups/Chin-Ups: Great for the back and biceps.

2. Isolation Movements:

BEGINNER'S BODYBUILDING

- Bicep Curls: For building bicep muscles.
- Tricep Extensions: Targets the triceps.
- Lunges: Helps with leg development.
- Dumbbell Rows: Focuses on the upper back.

3. Core Exercises:

- Planks: Strengthen your core.
- Russian Twists: Work on obliques.
- Leg Raises: Target lower abs.

4. Cardio: Include some cardiovascular exercise for overall fitness and calorie burning.

Don't forget to start with light weights to learn proper form and prevent injury. Gradually increase the weight and intensity as you progress. It's also essential to have a balanced diet and get enough rest for recovery. Consider consulting with a fitness trainer or coach for personalized guidance.

BEGINNER'S BODYBUILDING

Chapter 4

CREATING YOUR WORKOUT PLAN

Creating a customized bodybuilding workout plan is essential for achieving your fitness goals. It involves careful consideration of your objectives, fitness level, and available resources. In this process, you'll design a structured routine that focuses on resistance training, nutrition, and recovery. This plan will serve as your roadmap to building muscle, increasing strength, and improving overall fitness. Let's explore the key steps to crafting an effective bodybuilding workout plan tailored to your needs and aspirations.

Creating a bodybuilding workout plan requires careful consideration of your goals, fitness level, and preferences. Here's a basic framework to get you started:

1. Set Clear Goals:
Define your specific bodybuilding goals, such as building muscle mass, increasing strength, or improving overall fitness.

2. Determine Training Frequency:
Decide how many days per week you can commit to working out. Most bodybuilders train 3-6 days a week.

3. Split Your Routine:
Consider a split routine where you target different muscle groups on different days. Common splits include:

- Push/Pull/Legs
- Upper Body/Lower Body

BEGINNER'S BODYBUILDING

- Chest/Back/Shoulders/Arms/Legs

3. Choose Exercises:

Select compound exercises (e.g., squats, deadlifts, bench press) to work multiple muscle groups and isolation exercises (e.g., bicep curls, tricep extensions) for specific muscles.

4. Set Reps and Sets:

For muscle building, aim for 3-5 sets of 6-12 repetitions per exercise. Adjust the weight to reach muscle failure within this range.

5. Plan Progression:

Gradually increase the weight or intensity over time to stimulate muscle growth. Progressive overload is key.

6. Include Rest Days:

Allow for rest and recovery days to prevent overtraining and muscle fatigue. These are essential for growth.

7. Cardio and Flexibility:

Incorporate cardio for cardiovascular health and flexibility exercises to maintain mobility.

8. Nutrition:

Follow a balanced diet with adequate protein, carbohydrates, and healthy fats. Consider consulting a nutritionist or dietitian.

9. Supplements:

Consider supplements like protein powder, creatine, and BCAAs if needed, but focus on whole foods first.

10. Recovery:

BEGINNER'S BODYBUILDING

Prioritize sleep, hydration, and post-workout recovery techniques (stretching, foam rolling) for optimal results.

9. Track Progress:
Keep a workout journal to record your exercises, weights, and progress. Adjust your plan as needed.

10. Consult a Trainer:
If you're new to bodybuilding, consider working with a personal trainer to learn proper form and technique.

Consistency is key in bodybuilding. Stick to your plan, stay patient, and make adjustments as you progress toward your goals. It's also important to consult with a healthcare professional before starting any new exercise program, especially if you have pre-existing health conditions.

SETTING UP A WEEKLY ROUTINE
Creating a weekly routine for beginner bodybuilding workouts can help you progress effectively. Here's a sample plan, but remember to consult a fitness professional for personalized guidance:

Day 1: Chest and Triceps
- Bench Press (3 sets of 8-10 reps)
- Dumbbell Flyes (3 sets of 10-12 reps)
- Tricep Dips (3 sets of 8-10 reps)
- Tricep Pushdowns (3 sets of 10-12 reps)

Day 2: Back and Biceps
- Deadlift (3 sets of 5-7 reps)
- Lat Pulldowns (3 sets of 8-10 reps)
- Barbell Rows (3 sets of 8-10 reps)

BEGINNER'S BODYBUILDING

- Bicep Curls (3 sets of 10-12 reps)

Day 3: Rest or Light Cardio

Day 4: Legs
- Squats (3 sets of 8-10 reps)
- Leg Press (3 sets of 10-12 reps)
- Lunges (3 sets of 10-12 reps per leg)
- Leg Curls (3 sets of 10-12 reps)

Day 5: Shoulders and Abs
- Military Press (3 sets of 8-10 reps)
- Lateral Raises (3 sets of 10-12 reps)
- Front Raises (3 sets of 10-12 reps)
- Planks (3 sets, hold for 30-60 seconds)

Day 6: Rest or Light Cardio

Day 7: Rest

Repeat this cycle weekly, gradually increasing weights and reps as you progress. Ensure proper form, rest between sets, and include a balanced diet for optimal results. Adjust as needed based on your goals and recovery capabilities.

SPLITTING MUSCLE GROUPS

Splitting muscle groups, also known as a split routine or split training, is a popular approach in strength training and bodybuilding. It involves dividing your workouts into specific muscle groups or body parts on different days of the week. This method allows for targeted focus and recovery of individual muscle groups, promoting muscle growth and overall

BEGINNER'S BODYBUILDING

fitness. Split routines can vary widely, catering to different goals and preferences, such as upper/lower splits, push/pull splits, or body part splits like chest and triceps, back and biceps, and more. The effectiveness of a split routine depends on your fitness goals, training experience, and the balance between volume and recovery.

Splitting muscle groups is a fundamental concept in strength training and bodybuilding. It involves dividing your workouts into specific days or sessions, each focusing on different muscle groups. This approach allows for more targeted training and adequate recovery. Here's a brief introduction to the concept:

1. **Purpose:** Splitting muscle groups helps you effectively target and stimulate different muscle groups during your workouts. It prevents overtraining and allows for better recovery between sessions.

2. **Types of Splits:**

- Bro-Split: In this traditional split, each day is dedicated to a single muscle group, such as chest, back, legs, etc.

- Push-Pull-Legs (PPL): This split divides workouts into pushing exercises (chest, shoulders, triceps), pulling exercises (back, biceps), and leg exercises.

- Upper-Lower Split: Alternates between upper body and lower body workouts, allowing more frequency per muscle group.

- Full-Body Split: Works all major muscle groups in a single session, typically done multiple times per week.

BEGINNER'S BODYBUILDING

3. Benefits:

- Targeted Development: You can focus on specific muscle groups, addressing weak points or imbalances.

- Recovery: Splitting allows adequate rest for worked muscles, reducing the risk of injury and fatigue.

- Variety: Different exercises and muscle groups can be trained on separate days, preventing boredom.

4. Progression: To see gains, it's crucial to progressively increase weights, reps, or intensity over time within each split routine.

5. Personalization: The choice of split depends on your goals, schedule, and fitness level. Beginners might start with a simple full-body routine, while advanced lifters often opt for more specialized splits.

Incorporating a well-designed split routine into your training regimen can help you achieve your fitness goals efficiently and effectively. Be sure to tailor your approach to your specific objectives and consult with a fitness professional for personalized guidance.

PROGRESSIVE OVERLOAD

Progressive overload is a fundamental principle in bodybuilding that's essential for beginners looking to build muscle effectively. It involves gradually increasing the demands placed on your muscles over time to stimulate growth. This can be achieved by lifting heavier weights, performing more reps, or increasing workout intensity. As a beginner, understanding and applying progressive overload will be key to your long-

BEGINNER'S BODYBUILDING

term success in bodybuilding, helping you steadily progress and avoid plateaus in your muscle-building journey.

Progressive overload is a fundamental principle in bodybuilding that involves gradually increasing the demands placed on your muscles to promote growth and strength gains. For beginners, here's how to apply it:

1. **Start with a Solid Foundation**: Begin with a well-structured workout routine that includes compound exercises like squats, deadlifts, bench presses, and rows.

2. **Consistent Training**: Consistency is key. Stick to a regular workout schedule, aiming for 3-4 times per week for each muscle group.

3. **Incremental Weight Increases**: Gradually increase the weight you lift as you become more comfortable with the current weight. Aiming for 5-10% increases is a good guideline.

4. **Progressive Repetitions**: Over time, aim to increase the number of repetitions or sets you perform for each exercise.

5. **Monitor Progress**: Keep a training journal to track your lifts, sets, and reps. This helps you ensure you're consistently pushing yourself.

6. **Focus on Form**: Maintain proper form to prevent injuries. If you can't perform exercises with good form, it's better to lower the weight.

7. **Mix It Up**: Periodically change your routine to prevent plateaus and keep your muscles adapting.

BEGINNER'S BODYBUILDING

Remember that nutrition and rest are equally important for muscle growth. Consume enough protein and calories, get adequate sleep, and allow time for muscle recovery. Consulting a fitness professional or trainer can also be beneficial, especially for beginners, to ensure you're following a safe and effective progressive overload strategy.

BEGINNER'S BODYBUILDING

Chapter 5

REST AND RECOVERY

Rest and recovery are fundamental aspects of bodybuilding that often receive less attention than intense workouts and nutrition. However, they are equally crucial for achieving success, especially for beginners. In this context, rest refers to getting enough sleep and allowing your muscles to heal, while recovery involves strategies to aid this process. Here's a beginner's introduction to rest and recovery in bodybuilding:

1. Importance of Rest: Rest is when your body repairs and grows muscles. During intense workouts, small tears occur in your muscle fibers. Proper rest allows these tears to heal and rebuild, making your muscles stronger and bigger.

2. Sleep: Quality sleep is essential. Aim for 7-9 hours of uninterrupted sleep per night. Sleep promotes the release of growth hormone, crucial for muscle growth and overall recovery.

3. Nutrition: Proper nutrition complements rest and recovery. Consume enough protein to support muscle repair, and include a variety of nutrients to aid overall health.

4. Active Recovery: Active recovery involves light exercises like walking or stretching on rest days. This helps improve blood flow, reduce muscle soreness, and promote recovery.

5. Hydration: Stay hydrated as it plays a vital role in muscle function and recovery.

BEGINNER'S BODYBUILDING

6. Listen to Your Body: Pay attention to your body's signals. If you're excessively sore or fatigued, consider taking an extra rest day.

7. Consistency: Consistent rest and recovery practices are key. Don't underestimate their role in achieving long-term fitness goals.

8. Avoid Overtraining: Overtraining can lead to injuries and hinder progress. Schedule regular rest days into your training plan.

9. Recovery Techniques: Techniques like foam rolling, massages, and contrast baths can aid recovery by reducing muscle tension and soreness.

10. Progress Tracking: Keep a training journal to monitor your progress and assess whether your rest and recovery practices are effective.

Everyone's body is unique, so it may take some time to find the right balance of rest and recovery that works for you. Be patient, stay consistent, and prioritize your body's need for recuperation to optimize your bodybuilding journey.

THE IMPORTANCE OF REST

Rest is crucial for beginners in bodybuilding for several reasons:

1. Muscle Recovery: After intense workouts, muscles need time to repair and grow. Rest allows for this process to occur, leading to muscle development and strength gains.

2. Injury Prevention: Overtraining can lead to injuries, especially for beginners who may not be familiar with proper form and technique. Rest days reduce the risk of strains and sprains.

BEGINNER'S BODYBUILDING

3. Hormone Balance: Adequate rest helps maintain a healthy balance of hormones like testosterone and cortisol, which are essential for muscle growth and recovery.

4. Mental Refreshment: Rest days provide a mental break from the rigors of training, reducing burnout and helping beginners stay motivated in the long run.

5. Sleep Quality: Quality sleep is essential for recovery and muscle growth. Rest allows beginners to prioritize sleep and ensure they are well-rested.

6. Immune System Support: Intense exercise can temporarily weaken the immune system. Adequate rest helps the body recover and maintain a strong immune system.

7. Adaptation: The body adapts to exercise during periods of rest. Beginners need time for their bodies to adjust to the demands of weightlifting and other exercises.

In summary, rest is a fundamental component of any effective bodybuilding program, especially for beginners. It promotes muscle growth, prevents injuries, supports overall health, and contributes to long-term success in building a strong, fit physique.

SLEEP AND ITS ROLE

Sleep plays a crucial role in bodybuilding, especially for beginners.

Here's why:

BEGINNER'S BODYBUILDING

1. Muscle Recovery: During deep sleep, the body repairs and rebuilds muscle tissue that gets stressed during workouts. This is essential for muscle growth, making quality sleep a key factor in your progress.

2. Hormone Production: Sleep is when the body releases growth hormone and testosterone, both of which are vital for muscle development, strength, and recovery.

3. Energy Levels: A good night's sleep helps maintain high energy levels, which are necessary for effective workouts and consistent training.

4. Immune Function: Adequate sleep supports a healthy immune system, preventing illness that could disrupt your training routine.

5. Mental Focus: Sleep enhances cognitive function and concentration, helping you stay motivated and focused on your fitness goals.

For beginners in bodybuilding, aim for 7-9 hours of quality sleep per night to optimize muscle growth and overall performance. Prioritize a consistent sleep schedule, a comfortable sleep environment, and relaxation techniques to ensure you get the rest your body needs to thrive in your bodybuilding journey.

ACTIVE RECOVERY TECHNIQUES

Active recovery techniques are essential for beginners in bodybuilding to optimize their training and overall fitness journey. Active recovery involves engaging in low-intensity exercises and practices on rest days or in between intense workouts. Its primary goal is to promote muscle recovery, reduce soreness, and enhance overall well-being.

BEGINNER'S BODYBUILDING

For beginners, active recovery can be a game-changer, as it helps the body adapt to the demands of weightlifting and resistance training. In this guide, we will explore various active recovery methods suitable for newcomers to bodybuilding, including stretching, light cardio, foam rolling, and proper nutrition. By incorporating these techniques into your routine, you'll be better equipped to maximize your progress while minimizing the risk of injury.

Active recovery techniques can help reduce muscle soreness and improve overall recovery. Here are some effective options:

1. Light Cardio: Engage in low-intensity activities like walking, cycling, or swimming for 20-30 minutes. This promotes blood flow to muscles, aiding in the removal of waste products.

2. Stretching: Perform gentle stretching exercises to improve flexibility and alleviate muscle tension. Focus on major muscle groups like hamstrings, quads, and chest.

3. Foam Rolling: Use a foam roller to massage and release tight muscles. This self-myofascial release technique can relieve muscle knots and improve mobility.

4. Yoga or Pilates: Incorporate beginner-friendly yoga or Pilates sessions to enhance flexibility, balance, and core strength. These practices can also reduce stress.

5. Hydration and Nutrition: Stay well-hydrated and consume balanced meals with a mix of protein, carbohydrates, and healthy fats to support recovery.

6. Sleep: Ensure you get adequate sleep, as it's crucial for muscle repair and growth.

7. Active Rest Days: On rest days, engage in light activities such as leisurely hikes or recreational sports to keep your body active without overexerting.

Listen to your body and gradually increase the intensity of these techniques as you become more experienced in bodybuilding. Always consult a fitness professional if you have any concerns or specific needs.

BEGINNER'S BODYBUILDING

Chapter 6

SUPPLEMENTS FOR BEGINNERS

If you're just starting out and looking to incorporate supplements into your regimen, it's essential to understand their role in helping you achieve your fitness goals. Supplements can complement a balanced diet and rigorous training routine, providing your body with the necessary nutrients and support for muscle growth, recovery, and overall performance. Remember, while supplements can be helpful, they should be part of a broader strategy that includes proper nutrition, exercise, and rest.

Here are some commonly used ones for beginners:

1. Protein Powder: It helps meet your daily protein requirements, which is essential for muscle growth and recovery.

2. Creatine: Proven to enhance strength and muscle mass. It's one of the most researched supplements for athletes.

3. BCAAs (Branched-Chain Amino Acids): These can aid in muscle recovery and reduce muscle soreness.

4. Multivitamins: Ensure you're getting essential vitamins and minerals for overall health and performance.

5. Fish Oil: Contains omega-3 fatty acids, which can help reduce inflammation and support joint health.

6. Pre-Workout Supplements: These can boost energy and focus before workouts. Look for those with ingredients like caffeine and citrulline.

BEGINNER'S BODYBUILDING

7. Glutamine: May help with muscle recovery and reduce muscle soreness.

Supplements are meant to complement a balanced diet, not replace it. Consult with a healthcare professional or nutritionist to determine which supplements are right for you based on your specific goals and needs. Also, focus on a consistent workout routine and proper nutrition for the best results in bodybuilding.

PROTEIN SUPPLEMENT

You're a beginner in bodybuilding and considering protein supplements, here are some key points to keep in mind:

1. Whole Foods First: Before turning to supplements, focus on getting your protein from whole food sources like lean meats, poultry, fish, eggs, dairy, beans, and legumes. These provide essential nutrients and are generally more satiating.

2. Whey Protein: Whey protein supplements are a popular choice for many bodybuilders. They are quickly absorbed and provide a complete source of protein. You can use whey protein shakes as a convenient way to meet your protein needs.

3. Protein Timing: Spread your protein intake throughout the day. Aim for a source of protein with each meal to support muscle recovery and growth.

4. Dosage: The recommended daily protein intake for most individuals is around 0.8 to 1.2 grams of protein per pound of body weight. Supplements should complement your diet, not replace it.

BEGINNER'S BODYBUILDING

5. Read Labels: When choosing protein supplements, read the labels carefully to ensure they meet your dietary preferences and needs. Look for products with minimal additives and low sugar content.

6. Consult a Professional: If you're unsure about which protein supplement to choose or how much to take, consider consulting a registered dietitian or a fitness professional who can provide personalized advice.

7. Stay Hydrated: Protein supplements can be dehydrating, so make sure to drink plenty of water when consuming them.

8. Track Progress: Keep a log of your protein intake and monitor your progress in the gym to assess whether you're meeting your goals.

Remember that while protein supplements can be a helpful tool, they should not replace a balanced diet. Focus on overall nutrition, proper training, and consistency in your bodybuilding journey.

Here are some protein supplements that are commonly used by beginners in bodybuilding:

1. Whey Protein: It's a fast-digesting protein and a popular choice for post-workout recovery.

2. Casein Protein: This slow-digesting protein is often taken before bedtime to support overnight muscle repair.

3. Plant-Based Protein: Options like pea, rice, or hemp protein are suitable for vegetarians and vegans.

BEGINNER'S BODYBUILDING

4. Mass Gainers: These supplements combine protein with carbohydrates and fats to help with muscle and weight gain.

5. Egg White Protein: A high-quality protein source derived from egg whites.

6. Collagen Protein: Supports joint and skin health in addition to muscle recovery.

7. Blended Proteins: These products combine different protein sources for a balanced amino acid profile.

Supplements should complement a balanced diet, and it's essential to consult with a healthcare or nutrition professional before starting any new supplement regimen.

CREATINE

Creatine is a popular supplement among beginners in bodybuilding. It can help improve performance and muscle growth. Here are some tips for beginners:

1. Understand What Creatine Is: Creatine is a naturally occurring compound found in small amounts in foods and synthesized by the body. It plays a crucial role in energy production during short bursts of intense activity.

2. Dosage: A common starting dose is 3-5 grams per day. Some people also do a loading phase of 20 grams per day (divided into 4 doses) for the first 5-7 days, followed by a maintenance dose of 3-5 grams per day.

BEGINNER'S BODYBUILDING

3. Timing: You can take creatine at any time of the day. Some prefer it pre-workout for an energy boost, while others take it post-workout to aid recovery. Consistency is more important than timing.

4. Mixing: Mix creatine with water or a non-acidic beverage for best absorption.

5. Stay Hydrated: Creatine can draw water into your muscles, so it's essential to stay well-hydrated to prevent dehydration.

6. Combine with a Balanced Diet: Creatine works best when combined with a balanced diet and a structured workout routine. It's not a substitute for hard work and proper nutrition.

7. Consult a Healthcare Professional: If you have any underlying health conditions or concerns, it's a good idea to consult a healthcare professional before starting any new supplement reregimen.

8. Monitor Progress: Keep track of your progress to see if creatine is helping you meet your bodybuilding goals. Everyone's response to creatine can vary.

Be aware that Supplements should complement a healthy lifestyle that includes proper nutrition, regular exercise, and sufficient rest. It's also crucial to prioritize safety and follow recommended dosages.

MULTIVITAMINS

Multivitamins are dietary supplements that typically contain a combination of vitamins and minerals. They are intended to provide a convenient way to supplement your diet with essential nutrients that you may not be getting enough of through your regular food intake. It's important to consult with a

BEGINNER'S BODYBUILDING

healthcare professional before starting any new supplement regimen, as individual nutritional needs vary, and excessive intake of certain vitamins and minerals can have adverse effects.

A comprehensive multivitamin can provide a baseline of essential nutrients. Some commonly used vitamins and minerals that are important for beginners in bodybuilding to consider:

1. Vitamin D: Important for bone health and overall well-being.

2. Omega-3 Fatty Acids: May help reduce inflammation and support joint health.

3. Creatine: Can enhance muscle performance and growth.

4. Protein Powder: While not a vitamin, it's crucial for muscle recovery and growth.

5. Branched-Chain Amino Acids (BCAAs): Can help with muscle recovery and reduce muscle soreness.

6. Zinc and Magnesium: Important for hormone regulation and sleep quality.

7. Calcium: For bone health, especially if you don't consume dairy products.

8. Iron: Essential for oxygen transport in the body and overall energy levels.

9. Vitamin C: Supports the immune system and collagen production.

BEGINNER'S BODYBUILDING

Before taking any supplements, it's essential to consult with a healthcare professional or a registered dietitian. They can help you determine your specific nutritional needs and recommend the right supplements for your bodybuilding goals and overall health. Additionally, remember that a well-balanced diet should be the foundation of any fitness regimen.

BEGINNER'S BODYBUILDING

Chapter 7

TRACKING PROGRESS

Tracking progress in beginner's bodybuilding is essential for setting and achieving your fitness goals. Here are some key ways to do it:

1. Keep a Workout Journal: Write down your workouts, including exercises, sets, reps, and weights used. This helps you track your strength gains over time.

2. Take Progress Photos: Regularly take photos from different angles to visually track changes in your physique. Compare these photos over weeks or months to see improvements.

3. Measure Body Stats: Track measurements like chest, waist, hips, arms, and legs. This can help you see changes in muscle size and fat loss.

4. Monitor Weight: Keep an eye on your body weight, but remember that fluctuations are normal. Focus on trends over time, not daily fluctuations.

5. Use Fitness Apps: Many apps can help you log workouts and track progress. They often include features like charts and graphs to visualize your improvements.

6. Record Strength Gains: Note when you increase the weights you lift or the number of reps you can perform. This is a clear sign of progress.

BEGINNER'S BODYBUILDING

7. Track Nutrition: Maintain a food diary to ensure you're eating enough calories, protein, and other nutrients to support muscle growth.

8. Set Specific Goals: Establish clear, achievable goals. Whether it's increasing bench press weight or losing body fat, having specific objectives helps you stay motivated.

9. Assess Energy Levels: Pay attention to how you feel during workouts. Improved endurance and reduced fatigue can be indicators of progress.

10. Listen to Your Body: Sometimes, progress isn't just about numbers. Pay attention to how you feel, your energy levels, and overall well-being.

Progress in bodybuilding takes time, so be patient and stay consistent with your workouts and nutrition. It's also a good idea to consult with a fitness professional or a personal trainer to create a customized plan and ensure you're on the right track.

KEEPING A WORKOUT JOURNAL.

Keeping a workout journal is a great idea for beginners in bodybuilding. Here's how you can start:

1. Choose a Notebook: Select a notebook or use a fitness app to record your workouts. Make sure it's easily accessible.

2. Set Goals: Define your fitness goals, whether it's gaining muscle, losing weight, or improving strength.

BEGINNER'S BODYBUILDING

3. Plan Your Workouts: Create a workout plan that includes exercises, sets, reps, and rest times. Start with basic exercises like squats, bench presses, and deadlifts.

4. Record Each Workout: Write down the date, exercises, weights lifted, sets, and reps for each workout session.

5. Track Progress: Regularly review your journal to track your progress. Note improvements in strength and changes in your physique.

6. Listen to Your Body: Pay attention to how your body responds to workouts. Record any discomfort, soreness, or injuries.

7. Nutrition: Consider adding a section for your nutrition, noting your daily meals and calorie intake.

8. Rest and Recovery: Include rest days in your journal to ensure proper recovery between workouts.

9. Adjust as Needed: Modify your workout plan based on your progress and goals. Gradually increase weights or try new exercises.

10. Stay Consistent: The key is consistency. Stick to your workout routine and journaling over time for the best results.

Patience is essential in bodybuilding, and your journal will help you stay on track and make informed adjustments along the way.

A 7 DAY WORKOUT PLAN JOURNAL

Here's a sample 7-day workout plan journal that you can use as a template to track your workouts:

BEGINNER'S BODYBUILDING

Day 1: Monday

Workout: Full-body strength training
- Squats: 3 sets of 12 reps
- Push-ups: 3 sets of 10 reps
- Bent-over rows: 3 sets of 12 reps

Cardio: 20 minutes of brisk walking

Day 2: Tuesday

Workout: Cardio and core
- Jogging: 20 minutes
- Planks: 3 sets of 30 seconds
- Bicycle crunches: 3 sets of 15 reps per side

Day 3: Wednesday

Workout: Upper body focus
- Bench press: 3 sets of 10 reps
- Pull-ups: 3 sets of 8 reps
- Dumbbell curls: 3 sets of 12 reps

Day 4: Thursday

Workout: Yoga or stretching
- Practice yoga poses or perform 30 minutes of stretching exercises to improve flexibility and reduce muscle soreness.

Day 5: Friday

Workout: Lower body focus
- Deadlifts: 3 sets of 10 reps
- Lunges: 3 sets of 12 reps per leg
- Leg press: 3 sets of 12 reps

BEGINNER'S BODYBUILDING

Day 6: Saturday
Workout: High-intensity interval training (HIIT)
- Jumping jacks: 3 sets of 45 seconds
- Burpees: 3 sets of 12 reps
- Mountain climbers: 3 sets of 30 seconds

Day 7: Sunday

Rest day: Allow your body to recover. You can do light activities like walking or gentle yoga if you prefer.

Use this journal template to record the details of each workout, including the number of sets and reps, the weight lifted, and any notes on how you felt during the workout. This will help you track your progress and stay motivated on your fitness journey. Remember to consult with a fitness professional before starting any new workout program, especially if you have any underlying health concerns.

MEASURING RESULTS

Measuring your progress in beginner's bodybuilding is important to track your gains and stay motivated. Here are some common methods to measure results:

1. Body Measurements: Regularly measure key areas like your chest, arms, waist, hips, and thighs. Changes in these measurements can indicate muscle growth or fat loss.

2. Weight: Keep track of your body weight, but don't rely solely on it as muscle gain may offset fat loss.

BEGINNER'S BODYBUILDING

3. Progress Photos: Take photos from different angles (front, side, back) under consistent lighting and conditions. Compare these photos over time to visually assess changes in your physique.

4. Strength: Track your strength gains by recording the weights and reps you lift in your exercises. Increasing your lifting capacity is a good indicator of muscle development.

5. Endurance: Monitor your stamina and endurance during workouts. If you can do more reps or lift heavier weights over time, it's a positive sign of progress.

6. Body Fat Percentage: Consider getting your body fat percentage measured periodically using methods like skinfold calipers, bioelectrical impedance scales, or DEXA scans.

7. Training Log: Maintain a training log to record your workouts, including exercises, sets, reps, and rest times. This can help you see patterns and make necessary adjustments to your routine.

8. Nutrition Tracking: Pay attention to your diet and nutrition. Keep a food diary or use a nutrition app to ensure you're meeting your calorie and macronutrient goals.

9. Recovery and Energy Levels: Assess how you feel outside of the gym. Improved recovery, increased energy levels, and better overall well-being can be indicative of progress.

10. Consistency: Ultimately, the most important measure of progress is consistency. Are you consistently following your workout routine and nutrition plan? Consistency is key in bodybuilding.

BEGINNER'S BODYBUILDING

Remember that progress in bodybuilding takes time, and it's essential to be patient and stay committed to your goals. Adjust your training and nutrition as needed based on your measurements and how you feel during your workouts. Additionally, consulting with a fitness professional or trainer can provide valuable guidance on measuring and achieving your goals effectively.

BEGINNER'S BODYBUILDING

Chapter 8

COMMON MISTAKES TO AVOID

Embarking on a journey into the world of bodybuilding as a beginner can be both exciting and challenging. While the promise of sculpting a stronger and more impressive physique is alluring, it's crucial to navigate this path with caution. Novices often stumble into common pitfalls that hinder their progress and potentially lead to injury. In this guide, I'll explore some of the most prevalent mistakes that beginners should be aware of and strive to avoid. By steering clear of these errors, you can set yourself on a more effective and rewarding path to achieving your bodybuilding goals."

Here are some common mistakes to avoid when you're a beginner in bodybuilding:

1. Lack of Proper Form: Focusing on proper form is crucial to prevent injuries. Learn the correct techniques for exercises and start with lighter weights to master your form before progressing to heavier weights.

2. Overtraining: Beginners often push themselves too hard, too soon. Allow your muscles to recover by giving them enough rest between workouts, typically 48 hours for the same muscle group.

3. Neglecting Nutrition: Diet plays a significant role in bodybuilding. Don't overlook your nutrition; ensure you're eating enough protein, carbohydrates, and healthy fats to support muscle growth and recovery.

4. Skipping Warm-Ups and Stretching: Warm-up exercises and stretching are essential to prevent injuries and improve flexibility.

BEGINNER'S BODYBUILDING

Spend time warming up before your workout and stretching afterward.

5. Ignoring Compound Exercises: Compound exercises like squats, deadlifts, and bench presses target multiple muscle groups and should be a staple in your routine. Don't focus solely on isolation exercises.

6. Inconsistent Training: Consistency is key in bodybuilding. Stick to a regular workout schedule to see meaningful progress.

7. Neglecting Recovery: Sleep is vital for muscle recovery and growth. Aim for 7-9 hours of quality sleep each night.

8. Overemphasizing Supplements: Supplements can be useful, but they should complement a balanced diet, not replace it. Focus on whole foods first.

9. Ego Lifting: Don't lift weights that are too heavy just to show off. Start with manageable weights and gradually increase as you progress.

10. Lack of Goal Setting: Set clear, achievable goals to track your progress and stay motivated. Whether it's gaining muscle mass, increasing strength, or losing fat, having goals will help you stay on track.

11. Ignoring Mobility and Flexibility: Maintain flexibility and mobility through stretching and mobility exercises to prevent muscle imbalances and injury.

12. Not Listening to Your Body: Pay attention to your body's signals. If you're in pain or overly fatigued, it's okay to take a break or adjust your workout.

13. Comparison to Others: Avoid comparing your progress to others. Everyone's body is different, and progress varies from person to person.

14. Impatience: Building a great physique takes time. Be patient and stay committed to your routine.

15. Skipping Cardio: Cardiovascular fitness is important too. Incorporate some cardio into your routine to maintain overall health.

It's essential to start slowly, learn the basics, and gradually progress in bodybuilding. Consider working with a trainer or fitness professional to help you develop a safe and effective workout plan tailored to your goals and needs.

Chapter 9

STAYING MOTIVATED

Staying motivated as a beginner in bodybuilding is crucial for long-term success. Building a strong foundation in fitness requires dedication and perseverance. In this journey, you'll face challenges, but by setting clear goals, tracking progress, finding inspiration, and maintaining a positive mindset, you can stay motivated and make steady gains in your bodybuilding endeavors.

BEGINNER'S BODYBUILDING

Finding inspiration for beginner's bodybuilding can be motivating. Here are some tips to help you get inspired:

1. Success Stories: Look for success stories of individuals who started as beginners and achieved their bodybuilding goals. These stories can provide motivation and show what's possible with dedication.

2. Role Models: Identify bodybuilders or fitness influencers who inspire you. Follow their journeys, watch their workouts, and learn from their experiences.

3. Online Communities: Join online forums, social media groups, or fitness communities where beginners share their progress, challenges, and achievements. Interacting with like-minded individuals can be motivating.

4. Workout Videos: Watch workout videos on platforms like YouTube. Many fitness trainers offer beginner-friendly routines and tips that can inspire you to start and stay committed.

5. Personal Goals: Set clear, achievable goals for yourself. Document your progress with photos and measurements, and celebrate small victories along the way.

6. Visualization: Imagine yourself achieving your bodybuilding goals. Visualization can help you stay focused and motivated.

7. Local Gym: Visit a local gym and observe other members, especially those who started as beginners. You'll see that everyone begins somewhere, and progress is possible.

BEGINNER'S BODYBUILDING

8. Personal Progress: Keep a workout journal to track your own progress. Seeing improvements over time can be a powerful motivator.

Bodybuilding is a journey that requires patience and consistency. Stay dedicated, and let inspiration fuel your commitment to your fitness goals.

SETTING MILESTONES

Setting milestones for a beginner's bodybuilding journey can help track progress and stay motivated. Here are some milestones to consider:

1. Initial Assessment: Start with a baseline assessment of your current fitness level, including measurements, body fat percentage, and strength benchmarks.

2. Strength Gains: Aim to increase the weight or repetitions in your exercises over time. For example, set a goal to lift a certain weight for a specific number of reps within a few months.

3. Body Composition: Monitor changes in body composition by tracking weight loss, muscle gain, and reductions in body fat percentage.

4. Nutrition Goals: Establish dietary goals such as daily calorie intake, macronutrient ratios, and meal planning.

5. Fitness Routine: Stick to a consistent workout schedule, gradually increasing the intensity and variety of exercises.

6. Recovery and Rest: Ensure you're getting enough rest and recovery to avoid overtraining and injury.

BEGINNER'S BODYBUILDING

7. Consistency: Celebrate the accomplishment of sticking to your fitness plan consistently for a specific period, like 3 months or 6 months.

8. Performance Milestones: Set targets for specific exercises or lifts, like achieving a certain bench press or squat weight.

9. Flexibility and Mobility: Improve flexibility and mobility through stretching and mobility exercises. Measure progress by tracking increased range of motion.

10.   Body Measurements: Continuously measure key body parts (e.g., chest, waist, hips, arms, legs) to see changes in muscle size.

Remember, these milestones should be realistic and tailored to your individual goals and capabilities. Consult with a fitness professional to create a personalized plan and ensure safe and effective progress in your bodybuilding journey.

CELEBRATING ACHIEVEMENTS

Beginner bodybuilders often celebrate their achievements in various ways to stay motivated and reward themselves for their hard work and progress. Here are some common ways they might celebrate:

- Setting Goals: Setting and achieving specific fitness goals is a common way to celebrate progress. These goals could include hitting a certain weightlifting milestone, achieving a particular body fat percentage, or mastering a new exercise.

BEGINNER'S BODYBUILDING

- Tracking Progress: Keeping a fitness journal or using a workout app to track progress can be rewarding. Seeing improvements in strength, endurance, or physique can be a cause for celebration.

- Cheat Meal: Enjoying a well-deserved cheat meal or treat is a popular way to celebrate milestones. It provides a mental break from strict dieting and allows for indulgence in a favorite food.

- New Gym Gear: Treating themselves to new workout clothing, shoes, or accessories can be a way to celebrate progress and stay motivated.

- Sharing Achievements: Sharing their accomplishments with friends, family, or fellow gym-goers can be a source of motivation and celebration. Social support and recognition can be powerful motivators.

- Photos and Comparisons: Taking progress photos at regular intervals and comparing them can be a visual celebration of the changes in their physique.

- Rest and Recovery: Sometimes, a celebration can be as simple as taking a rest day or scheduling a relaxing massage or spa day to reward the body for its hard work.

- Personal Rewards: Setting personal rewards for achieving certain milestones, such as a weekend getaway, a new piece of workout equipment, or a personal training session, can be motivating.

- Competitions or Events: Some beginners may choose to participate in bodybuilding competitions or fitness events to celebrate their achievements and showcase their progress.

BEGINNER'S BODYBUILDING

It's important for beginners to find celebrations that align with their fitness goals and maintain a healthy balance between hard work and rewarding themselves. Celebrating achievements can help maintain motivation and make the fitness journey more enjoyable.

BEGINNER'S BODYBUILDING

Chapter 10

FREQUENTLY ASKED QUESTIONS (FAQs)

Here are 50 frequently asked questions about bodybuilding:

1. What is bodybuilding?
2. How do I get started with bodybuilding?
3. What are the benefits of bodybuilding?
4. What's the difference between bodybuilding and powerlifting?
5. How often should I work out as a bodybuilder?
6. What's the ideal bodybuilding workout routine?
7. How do I build muscle mass effectively?
8. Can women do bodybuilding?
9. What is the best diet for bodybuilding?
10. How many calories should I consume for bulking or cutting?
11. What are the essential macronutrients for bodybuilders?
12. Do I need to take supplements for bodybuilding?
13. What's the importance of protein in bodybuilding?
14. What are the best protein sources for bodybuilders?
15. How can I increase my bench press strength?
16. How do I avoid overtraining in bodybuilding?
17. What is the best rep and set range for muscle growth?
18. How long does it take to see results in bodybuilding?
19. Can I build muscle without lifting heavy weights?
20. How do I target specific muscle groups?
21. What's the role of genetics in bodybuilding?
22. Should I use free weights or machines for muscle growth?
23. How can I improve my form and technique?
24. What are the common mistakes to avoid in bodybuilding?

BEGINNER'S BODYBUILDING

25.   How important is rest and recovery?
26.   What's the difference between compound and isolation exercises?
27.   Can bodybuilding help with fat loss?
28.   How do I measure my progress in bodybuilding?
29.   What's the ideal body fat percentage for bodybuilders?
30.   How can I prevent muscle imbalances?
31. What's the significance of a warm-up and cool-down?
32.   How do I set realistic bodybuilding goals?
33.   What is periodization in bodybuilding?
34.   Should I do cardio as a bodybuilder?
35.   What's the role of testosterone in muscle growth?
36.   How do I avoid muscle soreness and injuries?
37.   Can I build muscle on a vegan or vegetarian diet?
38.   What's the difference between bulking and cutting phases?
39.   How do I break through a plateau in muscle growth?
40.   What's the importance of hydration in bodybuilding?
41. Can I compete in bodybuilding competitions?
42.   How do I choose the right bodybuilding coach or trainer?
43.   What's the role of mental preparation in bodybuilding?
44.   How do I deal with bodybuilding-related stress?
45.   What supplements help with recovery and muscle growth?
46.   How can I stay motivated in bodybuilding?
47.   What's the best time to work out for muscle growth?
48.   How do I avoid overconsumption of supplements?
49.   What's the importance of sleep in bodybuilding?
50.   How do I transition from bodybuilding to maintenance mode?

These are just a few of the many questions that arise in the world of bodybuilding. Feel free to ask for more information on any of these topics!

ADDRESSING COMMON CONCERNS

BEGINNER'S BODYBUILDING

1. What is bodybuilding?
Bodybuilding is a sport and fitness activity focused on developing and sculpting one's muscles through resistance training, nutrition, and supplementation.

2. How do I get started with bodybuilding?
To start bodybuilding, you need a structured workout plan, a balanced diet, and consistency in training. It's also helpful to seek guidance from a trainer or coach.

3. What's the difference between bodybuilding and powerlifting?
Bodybuilding aims for muscle size and definition, emphasizing aesthetics, while powerlifting focuses on strength and lifting heavy weights in three main lifts: squat, bench press, and deadlift.

4. How often should I work out as a bodybuilder?
The frequency of workouts can vary, but most bodybuilders train specific muscle groups 3-6 times a week, allowing for rest and recovery.

5. What is a typical bodybuilding diet?
A bodybuilding diet includes lean proteins, complex carbohydrates, healthy fats, and plenty of fruits and vegetables. Meal timing and macronutrient ratios are also crucial.

6. Do I need supplements for bodybuilding?
Supplements like protein powder, creatine, and branched-chain amino acids can be helpful, but they're not mandatory. Whole foods should form the basis of your nutrition.

7. How long does it take to see results in bodybuilding?

BEGINNER'S BODYBUILDING

Results vary depending on factors like genetics and effort, but noticeable changes can often be seen within a few months of consistent training and nutrition.

8. Can women do bodybuilding?
Absolutely! Women can engage in bodybuilding and achieve impressive results in terms of muscle development and overall fitness.

9. What are some common mistakes to avoid in bodybuilding?
Common mistakes include overtraining, neglecting proper form, not getting enough rest, and relying too heavily on supplements.

10.   Is bodybuilding safe?
When done with proper form, technique, and under the guidance of a qualified trainer, bodybuilding is generally safe. However, injuries can occur if precautions are not taken.

Bodybuilding is a personal journey, and individual results may vary. It's essential to set realistic goals, stay consistent, and prioritize your health and safety throughout your bodybuilding journey.

BEGINNER'S BODYBUILDING

Chapter 11

CONCLUSION

Starting a bodybuilding journey as a beginner is an exciting endeavor that can lead to significant physical and mental transformations. It's essential to begin with a well-structured workout program, focus on proper form, and gradually increase weights to avoid injury. Nutrition plays a crucial role, with a balanced diet that supports muscle growth and recovery. Consistency and patience are key, as results take time. Lastly, remember that everyone progresses at their own pace, so stay motivated, track your progress, and enjoy the process of becoming a stronger, healthier you.

ENCOURAGEMENT

Encouraging a beginner bodybuilder can make a significant difference in their fitness journey. Here are my encouragements.

Congratulations on starting your bodybuilding journey! Remember, progress takes time, so stay patient and consistent. Every workout and healthy meal you choose brings you one step closer to your goals. Believe in yourself, and don't be discouraged by setbacks. You've got the potential for greatness within you – keep pushing, stay dedicated, and watch your strength and physique transform! □□□ ♂□